DR. SEBI COOKBOOK

Mouth Watering Recipes to Detox the Body, Cleanse Your Liver and Drastically Improve Your Health through the Dr. Sebi's Alkaline Diet-

2021 EDITION

Contents

INTRODUCTION..5

CHAPTER 1: RULES TO FOLLOW FOR DR. SEBI DIET 7

YOU MUST ONLY EAT FOODS LISTED ON THE DR. SEBI FOOD LIST 7

MUST-HAVE KITCHEN EQUIPMENT 8

CHAPTER 2: DR.SEBI ALKALINE DIET 10

WHAT ARE ALKALINE DIETS?..10

ALKALINE DIET SAFETY CONCERNS 11

ADVANTAGES AND DISADVANTAGES 11

CONTAINERS 12

BASIC FOOD STORAGE GUIDELINES 13

ALKALINE VEGAN COLD FOOD STORAGE CHART....................................14

SUPPLEMENTS 16

CHAPTER 3: FOOD LIST 18

HYBRID FOODS 18

DEAD FOODS 19

GENETICALLY MODIFIED FOODS AND ORGANISMS..................................19

DRUGS 19

LIVING FOODS 19

RAW FOODS 19

CHAPTER 4: BREAKFAST 22

HERBAL SMOOTHIE..22

PEACH MUFFIN 23

RASPBERRY, PEACH AND WALNUTS SMOOTHIE......................................24

MINERAL SMOOTHIE..25

TAMARIND CUCUMBER BREAKFAST DRINK..26

GREEN SMOOTHIE..27

CANTALOUPE SMOOTHIE 28

KAMUT PORRIDGE 29

APPLE PORRIDGE 30

Teff Porridge...31

Tomato Omelet...31

Veggie Omelet..33

Spelt Waffles..34

Coconut Waffles...35

Brazil Nut Cheese...36

CHAPTER 5: LUNCH...**37**

Macaroni and 'Cheese'..37

Basil Avocado Pasta..39

Jamaican Jerk Patties..39

Kamut Patties..42

Tomato & Greens Salad...43

Cucumber & Onion Salad..43

Apple Salad...44

Cauliflower Soup...44

Parsley Mushrooms...46

Baked Portobello Mushrooms...47

CHAPTER 6: DINNER..**48**

Chickpea Mashed Potatoes..48

Mushroom and Onion Gravy...49

Vegetable Chili..50

Spicy Tofu Burger...51

Special Pasta Ala Pepper and Tomato Sauce..52

Spicy Chilled Red Pepper Soup..53

Alkaline Sushi-Roll Ups...54

Quinoa and Hummus Wraps..56

Pine Nut and Garlic Sauce..56

Turmeric Curry and Roasted Cauliflower...57

Hearty Minestrone...59

French Onion and Kale Soup...60

Ginger-Maple Yam Casserole...61

LAYERED CABBAGE ROLL CASSEROLE 62

VEGETARIAN PIE 63

CHAPTER 7: DESSERT AND SNACKS 66

GRILLED WATERMELON 66

LIME SORBET 67

HOMEMADE PROTEIN BAR 68

COCONUT CHIP COOKIES 69

CHICKPEA TOFU 70

BANANA PIE 70

MANGO CHEESE CAKE 71

AVOCADO GAZPACHO 72

CHOCOLATE CRUNCH BARS 73

SHORTBREAD COOKIES 74

PEANUT BUTTER BARS 75

ZUCCHINI BREAD PANCAKES 76

CHOCOLATE AVOCADO MOUSSE 76

SWEET TAHINI DIP WITH GINGER CINNAMON FRUIT 77

ALKALINE RAW PUMPKIN PIE 78

CONCLUSION 81

Introduction

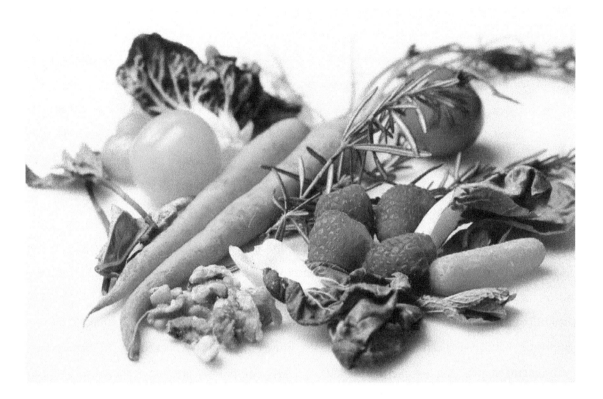

The food we eat today is unfortunately based on acidic foods, e.g. meat, dairy, sugar, etc. Today's diet is typically western, it is so high in processed ingredients, GMO and hybridized foods which unbalance the alkalinity of the blood. Dr. Sebi advised to avoid all these foods and eat only natural foods made by God. Dr. Sebi healing method revolves around the idea that disease exists only in an acidic environment. Therefore, his motto was: alkalize the environment and get rid of the disease. We know that the body constantly tries to maintain a healthy balance of 7.4 pH level in the blood. We can help it achieve and maintain this balance if we eat a natural alkaline based electric diet. Unfortunately, a typical western diet is high in very acidic foods. It is tasty, convenient, and nutrient deficient. Dr. Sebi protocol is based on the idea that the reason the western diet is unhealthy is that, being heavily processed, it lacks nutrition. That's why he insisted on foods that include over 100 minerals that support electrical activity and overall vitality of the body.

According to Dr. Sebi, most diseases are the result of acidity and mucus formation in the body, and he argued that diseases could be prevented or reversed when the body is given an alkaline environment. His healing program includes a strict dietary plan and supplements which claim to detoxify the body from many diseases and restore its alkalinity. The Dr. Sebi diet prohibits the use of all animal dietary products, and mainly focuses on vegetarian food intake, with far stricter rules than the vegan diet. For instance, it also prohibits the use of seedless fruits and only allows food that is on Sebi's approved list of vegetables: fruits, grains, etc. Due to its no animal food products approach, the Dr. Sebi diet is also known as the plant-based alkaline diet. The diet claims to rejuvenate the cells by allowing them to get rid of toxic metabolic waste. The diet is entirely made up of shortlisted foods, along with herbs and supplements. This diet also helps with conditions like AIDS, kidney disease, lupus, and other diseases. In fact, it can help reverse diseases. The treatments for these diseases require patients to eat natural grains, fresh fruits, and veggies, and refrain from animal-sourced food. The diet is naturally low in protein, so Dr. Sebi's supplements are important to keep up protein intake.

Through years of research and studies, Dr. Sebi found that diseases occur or can even grow when the mucus membrane of the cells and organs is compromised. For instance, if the bronchial tubes get too much mucus, then a person can be diagnosed with bronchitis. If the same mucus is produced and accumulates in the lungs, then a person is diagnosed with pneumonia. When the mucus moves to the pancreatic duct, then it can lead to diabetes. All of the compounds proposed by Dr. Sebi are extracted from natural plants, which make them alkaline. These compounds are important in reversing diseases that are only able to grow in acidic environments. The continuous use of all these natural remedies eventually detoxifies and cleanses the diseased body, and then brings it back to its natural alkaline state.

Chapter 1: Rules to follow for Dr. Sebi Diet

You must only eat foods listed on the Dr. Sebi Food List

Dr. Sebi insisted that you eat only the foods from his list of approved foods. Although the list is quite restrictive and many foods are left out, it contains wholly natural alkaline foods. Besides, Dr. Sebi insisted that no hybridized foods should be taken. By hybridized foods, he meant all the plants produced by artificial cross-pollination. Needless to say, most of the fruits and vegetables available today are hybridized.

Although Dr. Sebi diet seems rather restrictive, you can still create healthy, balanced, and tasty meals with the approved foods. One of the reasons so many foods have been left out from the list is that so much of what we eat today is hybridized. Dr. Sebi believed that hybridized fruits and vegetables generally are unnatural and not electric, and that their nutrient level is lower. One of the ways to know a plant that is hybridized is if it has no seeds. We now have quite a lot of seedless fruits ranging from watermelon, oranges, grapes, to tomatoes and berries. etc. Avoid these whenever you can. Dr. Sebi believed that natural foods are much healthier than those created by man.

To get the best out of Dr. Sebi's alkaline diet, he made certain rules and food principles which are expected to be followed by anyone interested in getting the results claimed from this diet. These rules though are very tough but they have proved effective. The rules are 8 in number and can also be found on Dr. Sebi's website. They include;

First Rule: Anyone who takes the alkaline diet must take only enlisted recommended foods outlined in the Dr. Sebi's nutritional guide.

Second Rule: Endeavor to drink a gallon of spring water every day (This is about 3.8 liters).

Third Rule: to take Dr. Sebi's supplements, it is advised that this should be done an hour before any other foreign medication is consumed.

Fourth Rule: A patient under Dr. Sebi's diet should not consume animal products of any sort.

Fifth Rule: Wheat products and are prohibited. Only natural growing grains (recommended in the guide) are accepted for consumption.

Sixth Rule: Alcohol is highly prohibited.

Seventh Rule: Canned food, a canned and seedless fruits are also prohibited.

Eight Rule: To get the best out of Dr. Sebi's cell food diet, it is advised not to microwave foods. According to the founder, "This kills the food and renders it ineffective"

Must-Have Kitchen Equipment

Most activities require certain tools and this also applies to cooking. Must-have kitchen equipment can be categorized according to its purpose.

1. **Cutlery**

These are spoons, knives, forks, ladle, spatula, tongs, slotted spoon, whisk, etc.

2. **Slicing tools**

Anything used for cutting, chopping, mashing or grinding falls into this category - knives, grater, potato masher, vegetable peeler, etc.

3. **Oven-safe storage containers**

There's nothing as convenient as taking your meal prep containers out of the refrigerator and right into the oven. Try to store your foods in different containers if they will require different methods of reheating. For example, a container of wild rice or quinoa would go straight to a steamer while my container of roasted chicken is placed in the toaster oven.

4. **A Crock-pot**

A great tool for lunch or reheating prepped meals.

5. **A Powerful Blender**

6. **A Food Processor of Juicer**

7. **A Toaster Oven**

8. **A Tea Kettle**

9. **Pans and Pots**

10. **Special extras (optional)**

These can help but you can easily do without them, e.g. spiralizer, an instant pot, air fryer, a tool for zesting key limes, steamer basket, sandwich maker, immersion blender, etc.

11. **Miscellaneous**

These are uncategorized items found in most kitchens, e.g. can opener, corkscrew, measuring cups or spoons, pepper mill, salad spinner, colander/strainer, cutting board, pots and pans, mixing bowls, etc.

Some of these tools are essential and no kitchen should be without them, e.g. cutlery, pots and pans, etc. Others, you should get if you can but there is no need to try and get them all at the same time. You can start by getting one or a couple from each of the categories and gradually add new ones if you think you need them. However, if you can't get most of these tools don't fret, our grandmothers prepared fantastic meals although they had very few pieces of cooking equipment and often did not even have electricity. Besides, what tools you'll need in your kitchen depends not only on your budget but also on the type of meals you are likely to prepare. For example, if smoothies are part of your diet, you will need a blender, if you bake often you will need kitchen scales, etc.

Chapter 2: Dr.Sebi Alkaline Diet

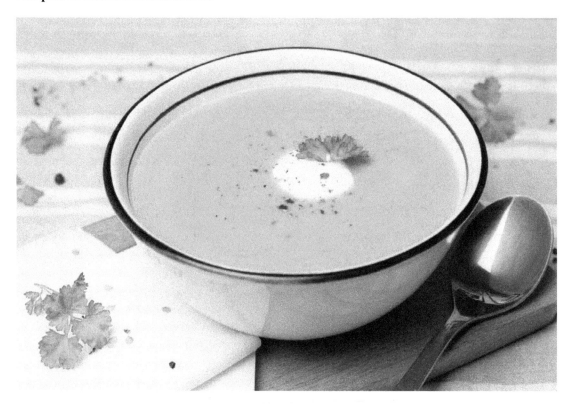

What are Alkaline Diets?

Alkaline diets are diets that are totally free from foods that contain acids. They are also termed electric foods, which help the body to naturally heal itself. They are naturally found in nature and are not modified, hybridized, and irradiated.

Alkaline foods are foods that assist in the increase of iron, copper, and other essential vitamins and minerals that make the immune system immuno-competent.

The meal prep basics revolve around preparing meals ahead of time and storing them in a way that will preserve their nutrients, flavor, and color. To achieve this, certain rules need to be followed. This diet is also known as "Dr. Sebi's cell food. It is a diet that is composed of plant-induced substances meant specially to regenerate the body cells. The cell food was created by a late Honduran herbalist known as "Alfredo Darlington Bowman".

It makes body regeneration possible by disposing of the contaminated wastes which are present in the body. It does this through introducing alkaline or non-acidic substances into the blood. This diet encourages the use of supplements (acknowledged). These supplements though limiting, costly, lacking in nutrients, it is said to promote healthy fitness.

The Alkaline diet is designed especially for a group of people. Anyone who desire to cure diseases or recover in overall health without using conventional drugs is advised to use the supplement pack and this cell food diet. To prove his stand on this, Dr. Sebi acclaimed that diseases will not live in someone whose body is induced with a lot of alkaline substances except the body becomes too acidic. Dr. Sebi's Alkaline is said to restore even an acidic body state and also cure life-threatening diseases like HIV/AIDS, sickle cell anemia, leukemia and lupus (though this was dismissed as false)

Alkaline Diet Safety Concerns

A lot of commentaries and opinions have been recorded on this. Dr. Sebi alkaline food diet is known to contain plant-based substances that can help keep the body fit under special conditions. This diet though does not have enough nutrients to keep the body fit because it is lacking in healthy protein foods which helps the body grow and replace worn out tissues and this makes the diet appear unsafe. The rules made to get results from this diet are very restrictive. Except a healthcare professional who will prescribe valuable supplements is contacted. Dr. Sebi's diet might not produce a healthy effect.

Avoid Hybrid Products

are foods that combine animal ingredients to plant-based ones. Hybrid products can be created when two varying fruits or vegetables are crossed to get a new variety. For example, in Dr. Sebi's diet, Kale and Brussels are part of the dietary list. When combined, they produce "kallets". This type of food blending is a vital tool that can be preferred if a person requires a change of diet. It helps to balance food gap. So many persons who are vegans may decide to try something new with the dairy products. It confuses people who engage in this diet as there is no base to follow (Mintel. 2017).

Advantages and Disadvantages

Why hybrid products are considered not good, there are benefits recorded on it. Some of them include;

Advantages

- It protects the body from many diseases

- These hybrid products cultivated under production are larger and do not consume much time in its growth process

- Hybrid products are said to protect the body from pests and other diseases

- It produces varieties of food species which are naturally not common.

Disadvantages

- Hybrid products come from different crossed products which certainly contain varying substances. These substances differ from the original one and most of these are dangerous to the body. They cause cancer.

- Hybrid foods do not use complex science and technology as genetically grown food

- They are less nutritious and have an entirely different taste from the original products

- During growth process, hybrid products require more water for irrigation.

Containers

Healthy food stored in the wrong way or wrong containers is a waste of time and money. As meal prepping is cooking for a few days or weeks, ahead, such meals are usually frozen or kept in the fridge. Either way, you need containers to keep the food in. Many different types of containers are available today and they come with different advantages, storing capacities, and prices. As proper storage can affect how a meal keeps and how it tastes, it's very important to choose containers that will help improve the taste rather than ruin it. But, before you go shopping for containers, make sure you know what you're going to use them for, e.g. for reheating, deep-freezing, pantry storage, etc.

11 common types of containers:

- Grab-and-Go containers

- Glass containers

- Stainless steel containers

- BPA-free containers

- Stackable containers

- Leak-proof containers

- Dishwasher-safe/Oven-safe containers

- Microwave-safe containers

- Freezer-safe containers

- Compartmentalized containers

- Airtight containers

Other things to consider when choosing containers is if you need reusable or single-use ones. Besides, containers are made from different materials which range from simple food plastic bags to sturdy ones made of plastic, silicone or stainless steel. However, most containers are made of plastic and if you are environmentally conscious, you can get some eco-friendly ones made from stainless steel, glass or bamboo. Personally, I like to go for over-safe glass containers. Although, they are pricey, the value you get from the investment is worth every penny. Another thing to consider is the shape and size. If you plan to store a huge amount of food or if you have very little freezing space, stackable containers would probably be the best. Alternatively, get some simple plastic food bags.

Basic Food Storage Guidelines

How tasty and healthy your frozen meals will depend not only on the ingredients used and your cooking methods but also on the way they were stored. Proper storage helps your meals retain as much of their natural flavor and nutrients as possible. So, knowing how to prepare meals is only half the job. They also need to be stored, frozen, defrosted, and reheated correctly. How long foods can be kept in a fridge or a freezer before their nutrients are affected, depends of the type of food but also on how they were processed. However, even deep-frozen foods cannot stay frozen indefinitely.

Alkaline Vegan Cold Food Storage Chart

Produce	Optimal storage temp (F)	Optimal storage temp C	Storage Life
Apples	30-40	-1 -4	1-12 months
Avocado, ripe	38-45	+3 - +7	
Avocado, unripe	45-50	+7 - +10	
Burro bananas, green	62-70	17 – 21	
Burro bananas, ripe	56-60	13 – 16	
Basil	52-59	11 – 15	
Beans, dry	40-50		6 – 10 months
Beans, green	40-45		7 – 10 days
Blackberries	32-33	0 – 1	2-3 days
Blueberries	32-35	0 – 2	
Cantaloupe	36-38	2 – 3	
Cherries, sour	32	0	3 – 7 days
Cherries, sweet	32	0	2 – 3 weeks
Cucumber	50-55		10 - 14 days

Currants	31-32		1-4 weeks
Lettuce	32	0	2-3 weeks
Figs	32-35	0 – 2	
Herbs	32-35	0 – 2	
Kale	32		2 – 3 weeks
Limes	48-55	9 – 13	
Mango	50-55	10 – 13	
Mushrooms	32	0	3 – 4 days
Peaches	31-32		2 – 4 weeks
Pears	29-31		2 – 7 months
Plums	31-32		2 – 5 weeks
Prunes	31-32		2 – 5 weeks
Squash	41-50		1 – 2 weeks
Strawberries	32	0	3 – 7 days
Turnip greens	32		10 – 14 days
Watercress	32		2 – 3 weeks
Tomatillo	55-70		4 – 7 days

SUPPLEMENTS

The supplement is an "all-inclusive package" that contains distinct products which cleanses the body, nourishes the cells and also returns it to its normal state at a fast rate. These supplements were recommended by Dr. Sebi and they include;

Banju: This is known to work for the nervous system condition. Example of ailments it handles includes; pain, irritability, stress and insomnia.

Bio Ferrocapsule: this is a blood purifier that contains herbs which are high in iron phosphate and some other mineral substances that aid nourishment of the body system.

Bromide Plus Powder/Capsule: this is a multi-mineral powder that is used in making nourishing shakes and teas. It helps the bones and thyroid gland. It also helps cure bad breath, pulmonary illnesses, respiratory problems, coughs etc. This supplement is known to contain zinc and calcium in high proportion.

Estro: This supplement is meant for the female endocrine reproductive system to maintain hormonal balance. This supplement also induces and helps in fertility. It heightens sexual appetite which may not have been in a woman previously.

Eye Wash: The function of this supplement is to cleanse the eyes and keep it back in shape.

Eva Salve: This supplement helps to tone the skin. It also gives the skin nourishment. It contains high calcium, fluorine and potassium phosphate. These minerals are known to help the elasticity of the skin.

Hair Follicle Fortifier: The function of this supplement is cleansing and making stronger the hair follicle to bring rise to new hair growth.

Green Food Plus*: This is a multi-mineral supplement that helps to promote good health. It offers "chlorophyll rich food" for the body performance.

Iron Plus*: This supplement is meant for blood nourishment. it also helps the brain and the central nervous system. This is specially made to curb issues of inflammation and it strengthens the body.

Testro*: This supplement helps to keep hormonal balance for the endocrine system. It helps to awaken sexual responsiveness in the male (an opposite of Estro).

Tooth Powder: it is used for cleansing the teeth and making it strong. It contains minerals and healing constituents that enables the teeth to be in good shape, whiten it and remove discolorations from the teeth.

Hair Food Oil: This nourishes the hair and also helps the scalp to be free of pesticide effects.

Chapter 3: Food list

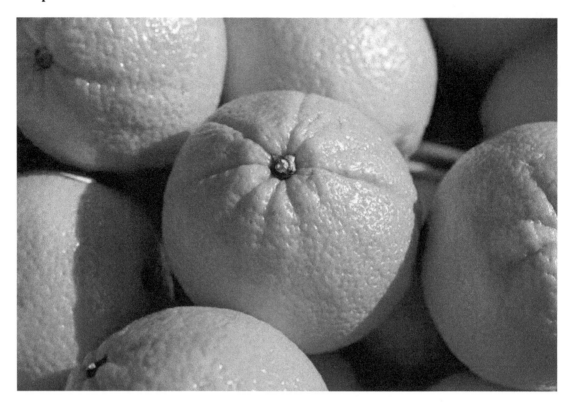

Dr. Sebi's method of classifying foods is different from any other method of food classification. He classified foods in the following ways: hybrid foods, dead foods, genetically modified foods, drugs, living foods, and raw foods.

Let me throw more light on each of Dr. Sebi's classification of foods.

Hybrid Foods

Hybrid foods are foods that have fewer amounts and/or no vitamins and minerals at all because they are cross-pollinated in their process of production.

They are not cultivated and grown in the wild. Hybrid foods are mostly sugars that cannot be identified by the body's digestive system. Some examples of hybrid foods are refined sugars, cows, pigs, chicken, sausage foods, and refined flour.

Dead Foods

Dead foods are overdone, over-processed, and toxic foods. They are foods that become toxic when they undergo the fermentation process and they have elongated life duration. Some of the examples of dead foods are synthetic foods, alcohols, deep-fried foods, sugars, cigarettes, refined foods, modified foods… and lots more.

Genetically Modified Foods and Organisms

Genetically modified foods and organisms are foods that are upgraded and developed by man genetically. These foods typically impair the immune system in the body.

These foods form unusual behavior in the body and also result in genetic problems. Some examples of genetically modified foods are foods that are developed hurriedly, such as brown rice, corn, yeast… and lots more.

Drugs

Drugs are consumables that are harmful to the body. Drugs cause your body more harm than good. They are exceedingly poisonous and acidic; hence, increasing the problems in the body.

Maximum numbers of drugs are extracted and synthesized. Some examples are prescription drugs, heroin, cocaine… and a lot more.

Living Foods

Living foods are foods that are not dead foods. They are foods that do not contain toxic constituents during the fermentation process.

Again, the constituents needed for the process of digestion is rooted in living foods which contain almost the same pH as water. Some of the examples of living foods are fruits, green vegetables, grains… and a lot more.

Raw Foods

Raw foods are living foods that are undercooked and have undergone processing. They are classified as foods that engage the use of sunlight for drying. These foods also comprise many constituents required for easy digestion and are damaged within a short time if not appropriately dried up.

Some examples of raw foods are dried fruits and vegetables, fermented fruit juice as well as roasted vegetables.

Below are Dr. Sebi generally approved List in the Nutritional Guideline. This list of vegetables, fruits, herbs, grains, oils and nuts and seeds is general and represents the general rule of thumb for foods to eat for healthy living. They include:

Dr. Sebi Food List Table

Vegetables	Fruits	Spices	Grains	Sweeteners	Her
Olives	Cantaloupe	Oregano	Kamut	Agave Syrup from cactus	Fennel
Wakame	Bananas	Cloves	Rye		Elderbe
Zucchini	Prickly Pear	Tarragon	Quinoa	Date Sugar from dried dates	Chamor
Wild Arugula	Peaches	Pure Sea Salt	Wild Rice		Red Ras
Cucumber	Soursops	Powdered Granulated	Amaranth		Tila
Mushrooms (but not Shitake)	Limes	Seaweed	Spelt		Ginger
Squash	Cherries	Cayenne	Fonio		Burdock
Onions	Plums	Habanero			
Garbanzo Beans	Berries	Sage			
Cherry and Plum Tomato	Tamarind	Sweet Basil			
Tomatillo	Rasins	Dill			
	Papayas	Basil			
	Soft Jelly Coconuts	Achiote			
	Currants	Savory			
	Apples	Thyme			
	Pears	Onion Powder			

Nori	Dates	Bay Leaf			
Turnip Greens	Figs				
Amaranth	Prunes				
	Orange				
Kale	Mango				
Okra	Grapes				
	Melons				
Watercress					
Dandelion Greens					
Chayote					
Arame					
Lettuce (but not iceberg)					
Bell Pepper					
Avocado					

Chapter 4: Breakfast

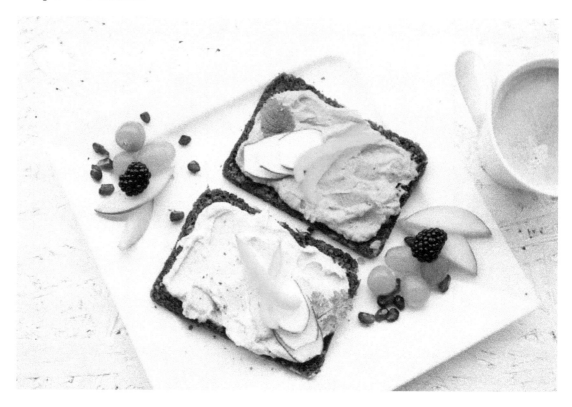

Herbal Smoothie

Prep & Cooking time: 5 minutes

Serving: 2

<u>Ingredients</u>

- 2 cups Dr. Sebi's Herbal Tea

- 1 burro banana, peeled

- 1 tablespoon walnut

- 1 tablespoon agave syrup

<u>Directions</u>

1. Plug in a high-speed food processor or blender and add all the ingredients in its jar.

2. Cover the blender jar with its lid and then pulse for 40 to 60 seconds until smooth.

3. Divide the drink between two glasses and then serve.

4. Storage instructions:

5. Divide drink between two jars or bottles, cover with a lid and then store the containers in the refrigerator for up to 3 days.

Nutritional Value per serving: 75.5 Cal; 2.1 g Fats; 0.9 g Protein; 13.2 g Carb; 1.8 g Fiber;

Peach Muffin

Prep & Cooking time: 25 minutes

Serving: 2

Ingredients

- 2/3 cup spelt flour

- ½ of peach, chopped

- 1 teaspoon mashed burro banana

- 2/3 tablespoons chopped walnuts

- 6 ½ tablespoons walnut milk, homemade

Extra:

- 1/16 teaspoon salt

- 2 2/3 tablespoon date sugar

- 2/3 tablespoon spring water, warmed

- 2/3 teaspoon key lime juice

Directions

1. Switch on the oven, then set it to 400 degrees F and let it preheat.

2. Meanwhile, peel the peach, cut it in half, remove the pit and then cut one half of peach in ½-inch pieces, reserving the other half of peach for use.

3. Take a medium bowl, pour in the milk, and then whisk in mashed banana and lime juice until well combined.

4. Take a separate medium bowl, place flour in it, add salt and date sugar, stir until mixed, whisk in milk mixture until smooth, and then fold in peached until mixed.

5. Take four silicone muffin cups, grease them with oil, fill them evenly with the prepared batter and then sprinkle walnuts on top.

6. Bake the muffins for 10 to 15 minutes until the top is nicely golden brown and inserted toothpick into each muffin comes out clean.

7. When done, let muffins cool for 10 minutes.

Nutritional value per serving: 76.1 Cal; 3.3 g Fats; 0.9 g Protein; 14.3 g Carb; 0.9 g Fiber;

Raspberry, Peach and Walnuts Smoothie

Serving: 2

Preparation & Cooking time: 5 minutes

Ingredients

- ½ of peach

- ½ cup raspberries

- 1 ½ tablespoons walnuts

- 2 tablespoons agave syrup

- ½ tablespoon Bromide Plus Powder

- 2 cups spring water

Extra:

- ¼ teaspoon salt

- 1/8 teaspoon cayenne pepper

Directions

1. Plug in a high-speed food processor or blender and add all the ingredients in its jar.

2. Cover the blender jar with its lid and then pulse for 40 to 60 seconds until smooth.

3. Divide the drink between two glasses and then serve.

Storage Instructions:

Divide drink between two jars or bottles, cover with a lid and then store the containers in the refrigerator for up to 3 days.

Nutritional Info: 165 Cal; 0.3 g Fats; 12 g Protein; 18.7 g Carb; 2.5 g Fiber;

Mineral Smoothie

Serving: 2

Preparation & Cooking time: 5 minutes

Ingredients

- 1 papaya, deseeded

- 3 dates, pitted

- 1 burro banana, peeled

- ¼ of key lime, juiced

- 1 tablespoon Bromide Plus Powder

Extra:

1 cup spring water

Directions

1. Plug in a high-speed food processor or blender and add all the ingredients in its jar.

2. Cover the blender jar with its lid and then pulse for 40 to 60 seconds until smooth.

3. Divide the drink between two glasses and then serve.

Storage instructions:

Divide drink between two jars or bottles, cover with a lid and then store the containers in the refrigerator for up to 3 days.

Nutritional Info: 152 Cal; 3.6 g Fats; 2.4 g Protein; 33 g Carb; 5 g Fiber;

Tamarind Cucumber Breakfast Drink

Serving: 2

Preparation & Cooking time: 5 minutes

Ingredients

- 2 cups Dr. Sebi's Herbal Tea

- 1 tablespoon tamarind pulp

- 1 cucumber, deseeded

- 2 ounces arugula

- 1 key lime, juiced

Extra:

- ¼ teaspoon salt

- 1/8 teaspoon cayenne pepper

Directions

1. Plug in a high-speed food processor or blender and add all the ingredients in its jar.

2. Cover the blender jar with its lid and then pulse for 40 to 60 seconds until smooth.

3. Divide the drink between two glasses and then serve.

Storage instructions:

Divide drink between two jars or bottles, cover with a lid and then store the containers in the refrigerator for up to 3 days.

Nutritional Info: 110 Cal; 0.5 g Fats; 2 g Protein; 30.5 g Carb; 6.5 g Fiber;

Green Smoothie

Serving: 2

Preparation & Cooking time: 5 minutes

Ingredients

- 1 cup dandelion greens

- ½ of cucumber, deseeded

- 1 apple, cored, deseeded

- 1 burro banana, peeled

- ½ tablespoon walnuts

Extra:

- ½ teaspoon Bromide Plus Powder

- 1 cup soft-jelly coconut milk

Directions

1. Plug in a high-speed food processor or blender and add all the ingredients in its jar.

2. Cover the blender jar with its lid and then pulse for 40 to 60 seconds until smooth.

3. Divide the drink between two glasses and then serve.

Storage instructions:

Divide drink between two bottles or jars, cover with their lids and then store the containers in the refrigerator for up to 3 days.

Nutritional Info: 317 Cal; 11 g Fats; 10 g Protein; 42 g Carb; 7 g Fiber;

Cantaloupe Smoothie

Serving: 2

Preparation & Cooking time: 5 minutes

Ingredients

- 1 cantaloupe, peeled, deseeded, sliced

- ½ cup Dr. Sebi Herbal Tea

- ½ of burro banana, peeled

- ½ cup soft-jelly coconut water

Directions

1. Plug in a high-speed food processor or blender and add all the ingredients in its jar.

2. Cover the blender jar with its lid and then pulse for 40 to 60 seconds until smooth.

3. Divide the drink between two glasses and then serve.

Storage instructions:

Divide drink between two jars or bottles, cover with a lid and then store the containers in the refrigerator for up to 3 days.

Nutritional Info: 114.7 Cal; 0.6 g Fats; 1.8 g Protein; 27.8 g Carb; 1 g Fiber;

Kamut Porridge

Serving: 2

Preparation & Cooking time: 15 minutes

Ingredients

- ½ cup Kamut
- ¼ teaspoon salt
- 2 tablespoons agave syrup
- ½ tablespoon coconut oil
- 2 cups walnut milk, homemade

Directions

1. Plug in a high-speed food processor or blender, add Kamut in its jar, and then pulse until cracked.
2. Take a medium saucepan, add Kamut in it along with salt, pour in the milk and then stir until combined.
3. Place the pan over high heat, bring the mixture to boil, then switch heat to medium-low level and simmer for 5 to 10 minutes until thickened to the desired level.
4. Then remove the pan from heat, stir agave syrup and oil into the porridge and then distribute evenly between two bowls.
5. Garnish the porridge with Dr. Sebi Diet's approved fruits and then serve.

Storage instructions:

Cool the porridge, divide evenly between two meal prep containers, cover with a lid, and then store the containers in the refrigerator for up to 7 days.

Reheating instructions:

When ready to eat, reheat in the oven for 1 to 2 minutes until hot and then serve with Dr. Sebi Diet's approved fruits.

Nutritional Info: 183 Cal; 2 g Fats; 10 g Protein; 30 g Carb; 4 g Fiber;

Apple Porridge

Preparation & Cooking time: *15 minutes*

Servings: *4*

Ingredients

- 2 cups unsweetened hemp milk

- 3 tablespoons walnuts, chopped

- 3 tablespoons sunflower seeds

- 2 large apples; peeled, cored, and grated

- Pinch of ground cinnamon

- ½ small apple, cored and sliced

How to Prepare

1. In a large pan, mix together the milk, walnuts, sunflower seeds, grated apple, vanilla, and cinnamon over medium-low heat and cook for about 3–5 minutes.

2. Remove from the heat and transfer the porridge into serving bowls.

3. Top with remaining apple slices and serve.

Nutritional Values :Calories 147, Fat 8.8 g,Carbs 17 g, Fiber 3.3 g ,Protein 3.2 g

Teff Porridge

Preparation & Cooking time: *30 minutes*

Servings: *2*

Ingredients

- 2 cups spring water
- ½ cup teff grain
- Pinch of sea salt
- 1 tablespoon agave nectar
- 1 tablespoon walnuts, chopped

How to Prepare

1. In a small pan, place the water and salt over medium-high heat and bring to a boil.
2. Slowly, add the teff grain, stirring continuously.
3. Now, adjust the heat to low and cook, covered for about 15 minutes or until the amaranth has thickened, stirring twice.
4. Stir in the agave nectar and remove from the heat.
5. Serve hot with the topping of walnuts.

Nutritional Values: Calories 215, Total Fat 2.9 g, Total Carbs 41.4 g, Fiber 6.8 g, Protein 6.9 g

Tomato Omelet

Preparation & Cooking time: *40 minutes*

Servings: *4*

Ingredients

- 1 cup chickpea flour

- ¼ teaspoon cayenne powder

- Pinch of ground cumin

- Pinch of sea salt

- 1½–2 cups spring water

- 1 medium onion, chopped finely

- 2 medium plum tomatoes, chopped finely

- 2 tablespoons fresh cilantro, chopped

- 2 tablespoons avocado oil, divided

How to Prepare

1. In a bowl, add the flour, spices, and salt and mix well.

2. Slowly, add the water and mix until well combined.

3. Fold in the onion, tomatoes, green chili, and cilantro.

4. In a large non-stick frying pan, heat ½ tablespoon of the oil over medium heat.

5. Add ½ of the tomato mixture and tilt the pan to spread it.

6. Cook for about 5–7 minutes.

7. Place the remaining oil over the "omelet" and carefully flip it over.

8. Cook for about 4–5 minutes or until golden-brown.

9. Repeat with the remaining mixture.

Nutritional Values: Calories 121, Total Fat 2.6 g, Total Carbs 18.8 g, Fiber 4.2 g, Protein 6.1 g

Veggie Omelet

Preparation & Cooking time: 20 minutes

Servings: 2

Ingredients

- ¼ cup chickpeas flour
- 1/3 cup spring water
- ¼ teaspoon fresh basil
- ¼ teaspoon dried oregano
- ¼ teaspoon onion powder
- ¼ teaspoon cayenne powder
- ¼ teaspoon sea salt
- ¼ cup plum tomato, chopped
- ¼ cup fresh button mushrooms, chopped
- ¼ cup green bell pepper, seeded and chopped
- ¼ cup onion, chopped
- 1 teaspoon grapeseed oil

How to Prepare

- In a bowl, add the flour, water, herbs, spices, and salt and mix well.
- In another bowl, mix together the tomato, mushrooms, bell pepper, and onion.
- In a skillet, heat the oil over medium heat.

- Place the veggie mixture in the skillet and spread in an even layer.

- Top with chickpea flour mixture evenly and cook for about 3–4 minutes.

- Carefully flip the omelet and fold it over.

- Cook for about 1 minute.

- Remove from the heat and serve hot.

Nutritional Values: Calories 83, Total Fat 3.2 g, Total Carbs 10.8 g, Fiber 2.3 g, Protein 3.4 g

Spelt Waffles

Preparation & Cooking time: 25 minutes

Servings: 3

Ingredients

- 1½ cups whole spelt flour

- 2 tablespoons date sugar

- 1½ tablespoons baking powder

- 1/8 teaspoon salt

- 1½ cups unsweetened hemp milk

- 1/3 cup grapeseed oil

- 1 teaspoon vanilla extract

Directions

1. In a bowl, add the flour, date sugar, baking powder, and salt and mix well.

2. Add the hemp milk, oil, and vanilla extract, and mix until well combined.

3. Set aside for about 3–5 minutes.

4. Preheat the waffle iron.

5. Generously grease the waffle iron.

6. Place 1/3 of the mixture into preheated waffle iron and cook for about 4–5 minutes or until golden-brown.

7. Repeat with the remaining mixture.

8. Serve warm.

Nutritional Values: Calories 547, Total Fat 30.3 g, Total Carbs 60 g, Fiber 8.2 g, Protein 9 g

Coconut Waffles

Preparation & Cooking time: *20 minutes*

Servings: *2*

Ingredients

- ¾ cup chickpea flour

- ¼ cup unsweetened coconut flakes

- 6–8 walnuts, chopped

- 1–2 tablespoon date syrup

- 1 tablespoon bromide mix

- Pinch of sea salt

- ½ cup unsweetened hemp milk

- ½ cup spring water

- ½ teaspoon vanilla extract

Directions

1. In a high-powered blender, put in all the ingredients and pulse until well combined.

2. Set aside for about 3–5 minutes.

3. Preheat the waffle iron.

4. Generously grease the waffle iron.

5. Place half of the mixture into preheated waffle iron and cook for about 4–5 minutes or until golden-brown.

6. Repeat with the remaining mixture.

7. Serve warm.

Nutritional Values:Calories 459, Fat 19.1 g Total Carbs 56.5 g   Fiber 15.6 g Protein 18.9 g

Brazil Nut Cheese

Preparation & Cooking Time: 5 minutes + soak time (2 hours)

Servings: 6 cups

Ingredients:

- Soaked Brazil nuts* (1 lb./450 g)

- Lime juice (half of 1 lime)

- Sea salt (2 tsp.)

- Cayenne (.5 tsp.)

- Onion powder (1 tsp.)

- Hemp milk (1.5 cups)

- Spring Water (1.5 cups)

- Grapeseed oil (2 tsp.)

- Food processor or blender also needed

Directions

1. It is recommended to soak the nuts overnight, but two hours will suffice.

2. Toss all of the fixings into the blender (minus the water).

3. Slowly begin by adding ½ cup of water to combine the fixings (2 min.).

4. Continue adding water (½ cup), blending until the preferred texture is attained.

Chapter 5: Lunch

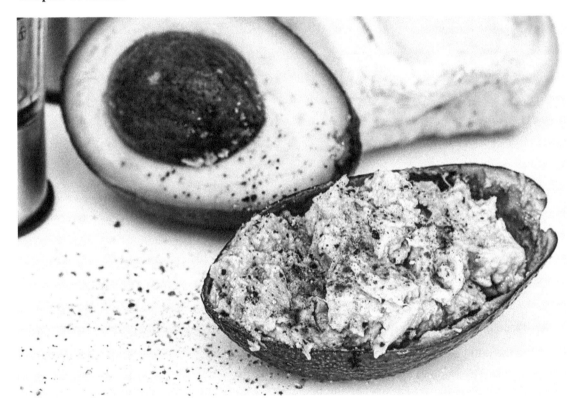

Macaroni and 'Cheese'

Preparation & Cooking Time: 70 minutes

Servings: 8-10

Ingredients:

- 12 ounces any alkaline pasta

- 1/4 cup chickpea flour

- 1 cup raw Brazil nuts

- 1/2 teaspoon ground achiote

- 2 teaspoons onion powder

- 1 teaspoon pure sea salt

- 2 teaspoons grapeseed oil

- 1 cup homemade hemp seed milk

- 1 cup spring water + extra for soaking

- Juice from 1/2 key lime

Directions:

1. Put the Brazil nuts in a medium bowl and cover them with spring water. Soak overnight.

2. Cook your favorite alkaline pasta.

3. Preheat your oven to 350 degrees Fahrenheit.

4. Place the cooked pasta in a baking dish and drizzle extra grapeseed oil to prevent it from sticking to the bottom.

5. Add all ingredients to a blender and blend for 2 to 4 minutes until smooth.

6. Pour the Brazil nut sauce over the macaroni and mix well.

7. Put the baking dish in the oven and bake for about 30 minutes.

8. Serve and enjoy your Macaroni and 'Cheese'!

Nutrition: Calories: 360 kcal. Fat: 6g. Carbs: 13.4g. Protein: 22.5g.

Basil Avocado Pasta

Preparation & Cooking Time: 30 minutes

Servings: 4

Ingredients:

• 4 cups cooked spelt pasta

• 1 medium diced avocado

• 2 cups halved cherry tomatoes

• 1 minced fresh basil

• 1 teaspoon agave syrup

• 1 tablespoon key lime juice

• 1/4 cup olive oil

Directions:

1. Place the cooked pasta in a large bowl.

2. Add halved cherry tomatoes, and diced avocado.

3. Whisk olive oil, agave syrup,and pure sea salt, and key lime juice in a separate bowl.

4. Pour it over the pasta and stir until well combined.

5. Enjoy your Basil Avocado Pasta!

Nutrition: Calories: 458kcal. Fat: 7g. Carbs: 22g.   Protein: 18g.

Jamaican Jerk Patties

Preparation & Cooking Time: 1 hour & 35 minutes

Servings: 3-4

Ingredients:

Filling:

- 1 cup cooked garbanzo beans

- 1/2 cup diced green pepper

- 1 chopped plum tomato

- 2 cups chopped mushrooms

- 1 cup chopped butternut squash

- 1/2 cup diced onions

- 1 tablespoon onion powder

- 1 teaspoon ginger

- 2 teaspoons thyme

- 1 tablespoon agave syrup

- 1/2 teaspoon cayenne powder

- 1 teaspoon allspice

- 1/4 teaspoon cloves

- 1 teaspoon pure sea salt

Crust:

- 1 1/2 cups spelt flour

- 1/4 cup aquafaba

- 1 teaspoon pure sea salt

- 1/8 teaspoon ginger powder

- 1 teaspoon onion powder

- 1 tablespoon grapeseed oil

- 1 cup spring water

Directions:

1. Preheat your oven to 350 degrees Fahrenheit.

2. Add all vegetables, excluding cherry tomatoes, to a food processor. Pulse a few times to chop them into large pieces.

3. Mix blended vegetables with seasonings and tomatoes in a large bowl. This constitutes the filling for the patties.

4. In a separate large bowl, combine the spelt flour, grapeseed oil, and seasonings.

5. Pour in 1/2 cup of spring water and knead the dough into a ball, adding more water or flour as needed.

6. Leave the dough to rest for 5 to 10 minutes. Knead again for a few minutes, then divide it into 8 equal parts.

7. Make each part into a ball and roll each ball out into a 6 to 7-inch circle.

8. Take a dough circle and place 1/2 cup of the filling in the center. Brush all edges of the dough with aquafaba, fold it over in half, and seal the edges together with a fork.

9. Repeat step 8 until all the dough circles are filled.

10. Lightly coat a baking sheet with a little grapeseed oil.

11. Bake filled patties for about 25 to 30 minutes until golden brown.

12. Serve and enjoy your Jamaican Jerk Patties!

Nutrition: Calories: 375kcal. Fat: 2g. Carbs: 5g. Protein: 8g.

Kamut Patties

Preparation & Cooking Time: 45 minutes

Servings: 3-4

Ingredients:

• 3 cups cooked kamut cereal

• 1 cup minced red onions

• 1 cup chopped yellow & green peppers

• 1 cup spelt flour

• ½ cup homemade hemp seed milk (see recipe)

• 1 tablespoon basil

• ½ teaspoon cayenne powder

• 1 tablespoon oregano

• 1 tablespoon onion powder

• 1 teaspoon pure sea salt

• 2 tablespoons grade seed oil

Directions:

1. Combine vegetables, hempseed milk, seasonings, and kamut cereal in a large bowl.

2. Put 1/2 cup of spelt flour in the bowl and mix it well. Continue adding more flour until it can be formed into patties.

3. Warm the grapeseed oil in a skillet on medium heat. Form patties from the mixture and place them on the pan.

4. Cook patties for about 4 to 5 minutes on each side.

5. Serve and enjoy your Kamut Patties!

Nutrition: Calories: 412kcal. Fat: 7g. Carbs: 12g. Protein: 15g.

Tomato & Greens Salad

Preparation & Cooking Time: 10 minutes

Servings: 4

Ingredients:

• 6 cups fresh baby greens

• 3 cups cherry tomatoes

• 2 tablespoons extra-virgin olive oil

• 1 tablespoon fresh lemon juice

Directions:

In a large bowl, add all ingredients and toss to coat well.

Serve immediately.

Nutrition: Calories: 90 kcal. Total Fat: 7.3g. Total Carbs: 6.3g. Fiber: 2.2g. Protein: 1.7g.

Cucumber & Onion Salad

Preparation & Cooking Time: 10 minutes

Servings: 5

Ingredients:

• 3 large cucumbers, sliced thinly

• ½ cup onion, sliced

• 2 tablespoons olive oil

- 1 tablespoon fresh apple cider vinegar

- Sea salt, to taste

- ¼ cup fresh cilantro, chopped

Directions:

In a large bowl, add all ingredients and toss to coat well.

Serve immediately.

Nutrition: Calories: 81 kcal.   Total Fat: 5.8g.   Total Carbs: 7.7g.   Fiber: 1.2g.   Protein: 1.3g.

Apple Salad

Preparation & Cooking Time: 10 minutes

Servings: 4

Ingredients:

- 4 large apples, cored and sliced

- 6 cups fresh baby spinach

- 3 tablespoons extra-virgin olive oil

- 2 tablespoons apple cider vinegar

Directions:

In a large bowl, add all the ingredients and toss to coat well.

Serve immediately.

Nutrition: Calories: 218 kcal.   Total Fat: 11.1g.   Total Carbs: 32.5g.   Fiber: 6.4g.   Protein: 1.9g.

Cauliflower Soup

Preparation & Cooking Time: 35 minutes

Servings: 4

Ingredients:

• 2 tablespoons olive oil

• 1 yellow onion, chopped

• 2 carrots, peeled and chopped

• 2 celery stalks, chopped

• 2 garlic cloves, minced

• 1 Serrano pepper, chopped finely

• 1 teaspoon ground turmeric

• 1 teaspoon ground coriander

• 1 teaspoon ground cumin

• ¼ teaspoon red pepper flakes, crushed

• 1 head cauliflower, chopped

• 4 cups vegetable broth

• 1 cup coconut milk

• Sea salt and freshly ground black pepper, to taste

• 2 tablespoons fresh chives, chopped

Directions:

1. In a large saucepan, heat the oil over medium heat and sauté the onion, carrot, and celery for 5-6 minutes.

2. Add the garlic, Serrano pepper, and spices and sauté for about 1 minute.

3. Add the cauliflower and cook for 5 minutes, stirring occasionally.

4. Add the broth and coconut milk and bring to a boil over medium-high heat.

5. Reduce the heat to low and simmer for 15 minutes.

6. Season the soup with salt and black pepper and remove from the heat.

7. Serve hot with a topping of chives.

Nutrition: Calories 285 kcal.   Total Fat: 23g.   Total Carbs: 14.9g.   Fiber: 4.8g.   Protein: 8.5g.

Parsley Mushrooms

Preparation & Cooking Time: 29 minutes

Servings: 2

Ingredients:

• 2 tablespoons olive oil

• 2-3 tablespoons onion, minced

• ½ teaspoon garlic, minced

• 12 ounces fresh mushrooms, sliced

• 1 tablespoon fresh parsley

• Sea salt and freshly ground black pepper, to taste

Directions:

In a skillet, heat the oil over medium heat and sauté the onion and garlic for 2-3 minutes.

Add the mushrooms and cook for 8-10 minutes or until desired doneness.

Stir in the parsley, salt and black pepper and remove from the heat.

Serve hot.

Nutrition: Calories: 162 kcal.   Total Fat: 14.5g.   Total Carbs: 6.9g.   Fiber: 2g.   Protein: 5.6g.

Baked Portobello Mushrooms

Preparation & Cooking time: 40 minutes

Serving: 2

Ingredients

- 2 caps of Portobello mushrooms, destemmed
- 2/3 teaspoon minced sage
- 2/3 teaspoon thyme
- 2/3 tablespoon key lime juice

Extra:

- 2 tablespoons alkaline soy sauce

Directions

1. Switch on the oven, then set it to 400 degrees F and let it preheat.
2. Take a baking dish and then arrange mushroom caps in it, cut side up.
3. Take a small bowl, place remaining ingredients in it, stir until mixed, brush the mixture over inside and outside mushrooms, and then let them marinate for 15 minutes.
4. Bake the mushrooms for 30 minutes, flipping halfway.
5. Storage instructions:
6. Cool the mushrooms, divide evenly between two meal prep containers, cover with a lid, and then store the containers in the refrigerator for up to 7 days.

Reheating instructions:

When ready to eat, reheat in the oven for 1 to 2 minutes until hot and then serve.

Nutritional Info: 72 Cal; 2 g Fats; 6 g Protein; 10 g Carb; 2 g Fiber;

Chapter 6: Dinner

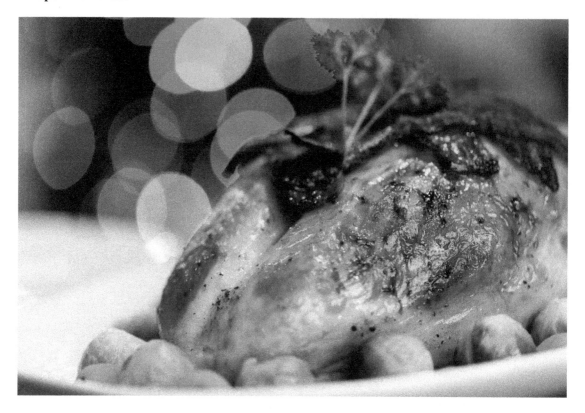

Chickpea Mashed Potatoes

Preparation & Cooking Time: 35 minutes

Servings: 4

Ingredients

- 2 cups chickpeas, cooked

- ¼ cup green onions, diced

- 2 teaspoons sea salt

- 2 teaspoons onion powder

- 1 cup walnut milk; homemade, unsweetened

Directions

1. Plug in a food processor, add chickpeas to it, pour in the milk, and then add salt and onion powder.

2. Cover the blending jar with its lid and then pulse for 1 to 2 minutes until smooth; blend in water if the mixture is too thick.

3. Take a medium saucepan, place it over medium heat, and then add blended chickpea mixture in it.

4. Stir green onions into the chickpeas mixture and then cook the mixture for 30 minutes, stirring constantly. Serve straight away.

Nutrition: 145.8 Calories 19.1g Carbs 7.3g Fat 3.3g Protein

Mushroom and Onion Gravy

Preparation & Cooking Time: 23 minutes

Servings: 4

Ingredients

- 1 cup sliced onions, chopped

- 1 cup mushrooms, sliced

- 2 teaspoons onion powder

- 2 teaspoons sea salt

- 1 teaspoon dried thyme

- 6 tablespoons chickpea flour

- ½ teaspoon cayenne pepper

- 1 teaspoon dried oregano

- 4 tablespoons grapeseed oil

- 4 cups spring water

Directions

1. Take a medium pot, place it over medium-high heat, add oil and when hot, add onions and mushrooms, and then cook for 1 minute.

2. Season the vegetables with onion powder, salt, thyme, and oregano. Stir until mixed, and cook for 5 minutes. Pour in water, stir in cayenne pepper, stir well, and then bring the mixture to a boil. Slowly stir in chickpea flour, and bring the mixture to a boil again.

3. Remove pan from heat and then serve gravy with a favorite dish.

Nutrition: 120 Calories 8.4g Carbs 7.6g Fat 2.2g Protein

Vegetable Chili

Prep & Cooking time: 35 minutes

Servings: 6

Ingredients

- 2 cups black beans, cooked

- 1 medium red bell pepper; deseeded, chopped

- 1 poblano chili; deseeded, chopped

- 2 jalapeño chilies; deseeded, chopped

- 4 tablespoons cilantro, chopped

- 1 large white onion; peeled, chopped

- 1 ½ tablespoon minced garlic

- 1 ½ teaspoon sea salt

- 1 ½ teaspoon cumin powder

- 1 ½ teaspoon red chili powder

- 3 teaspoons lime juice

- 2 tablespoons grapeseed oil

- 2 ½ cups vegetable stock

Directions

1. Take a large pot, place it over medium-high heat, add oil and when hot, add onion and cook for 4–5 minutes until translucent. Add bell pepper, jalapeno pepper, poblano chili, and garlic and then cook for 3–4 minutes until veggies turn tender.

2. Season the vegetables with salt, stir in cumin powder and red chili powder, then add chickpeas and pour in vegetable stock. Bring the mixture to a boil, then switch heat to medium-low and simmer the chili for 15–20 minutes until thickened slightly.

3. Then remove the pot from heat, ladle chili stew among six bowls, drizzle with lime juice, garnish with cilantro, and serve.

Nutrition: 224.2 Calories 42.6g Carbs 1.2g Fat 12.5g Protein

Spicy Tofu Burger

Preparation & Cooking Time: 20 minutes

Servings: 4

Ingredients

- 500g of firm tofu

- 100g of green bell pepper

- 6 teaspoon of organic chili sauce

- ½ a teaspoon of sea salt

- 2 teaspoon of extra virgin olive oil

- Pepper as needed

Directions

1. Chop up the tofu, bell peppers and onions into tiny pieces. Take a pan and place it over medium heat

2. Add oil and heat it up, add the cut veggies and stir fry for 5 minutes. Add tofu and stir fry for another 15 minutes. Add chili sauce into the mix and season with some pepper and salt to adjust the flavor accordingly

3. Add water and wet the mixture. Serve with alkaline bread, keeping the mixture between two pieces of bread

Nutrition 496 Calories 13g Fats 74g Carbs 6g Fiber

Special Pasta Ala Pepper and Tomato Sauce

Preparation & Cooking Time: 15 minutes

Servings: 4

Ingredients

- 500g of vegetable pasta

- 300g of tomatoes

- ½ a cup of sun-dried tomatoes

- 1 small sized red bell pepper

- 1 small sized Zucchini

- 1 piece of onion

- 2 pieces of garlic cloves

- 1 piece of chili

- 5 pieces of fresh basil leaves

- 2-3 tablespoon of cold pressed olive oil

- Sea salt as needed

- Pepper as needed

Directions

1. Cook the pasta properly according to the specified package instructions. Cut up the tomatoes, bell pepper, zucchini into fine cubes and chop the chili, garlic, and onions. Take a pan and place it over medium heat

2. Add oil and heat up the oil. Add onions, chili, pepper, and garlic and fry them for a few minutes

3. Add tomatoes, zucchini and cook for 5-10 minutes more. Add basil

4. Season with pepper and salt to adjust the flavor

5. Add pasta on top your serving plate

6. Pour the sauce and season Serve!

Nutrition 591 Calories 22g Fats 73g Carbs

Spicy Chilled Red Pepper Soup

Preparation & Cooking Time: 45 minutes

Servings: 4

Ingredients:

- 1 teaspoon avocado oil

- ¼ cup diced onions

- 2 garlic cloves, crushed

- 2 cups diced red bell peppers

- 2 cups vegetable broth

- ½ to 1 jalapeño, seeded and diced

- 1 teaspoon sea salt

- ½ cup small-diced red bell peppers

- ½ cup small-diced yellow bell peppers

Directions:

1. To a skillet over medium-high heat, add the avocado oil, onions, garlic, and red bell peppers, and sauté for 2 to 3 minutes, or until the onions are soft; allow to cool.

2. In a blender, blend together the sautéed mixture, vegetable broth, jalapeño, and salt until everything is well combined and completely liquid; adjust seasonings to your preference.

3. Transfer the soup to a medium bowl, and stir in the diced red and yellow bell peppers.

4. Cover and refrigerate for 20 to 30 minutes to cool or chill overnight.

5. Ladle into 2 large or 4 small bowls and enjoy.

Nutrition: 225 calories 18g fiver 25g protein

Alkaline Sushi-Roll Ups

Preparation & Cooking Time: 35 minutes

Servings: 2

Ingredients:

For hummus

- 1 Clove of garlic

- ½ Lemon juice

- Almonds handful

- 1 pinch Cumin

- 1 pinch Himalayan salt

- A glug Olive oil

- 1 tsp Tahini

- 100g Chickpeas

For the roll-ups:

- 1 Cucumber

- 2 Zucchini/Courgette

- 1 Carrot

- 1 Capsicum

- 1 small Coriander/cilantro

- 1 Avocado

Directions:

For the Hummus

1. All you have to do is to get a food processor or blender. Blend until everything is smooth.

2. Then add some more lemon or olive oil to suit your taste.

For the Alkaline Sushi Roll-Ups

1. Cut off both ends of the Zucchini Use a vegetable peeler to peel it into thin, long strips

2. Lay out the zucchini strip and spread the almond hummus on it

3. Add some matchsticks of avocado, veggies and a few pieces of coriander. Spray some of the sesame seeds on top. Roll and enjoy

Nutrition: 158 calories 10g fiber 9g fats

Quinoa and Hummus Wraps

Preparation & Cooking Time: 12 minute

Servings: 4

<u>Ingredients</u>:

- 1 cup Quinoa

- 1 cup Hummus

- 1 cup Avocado

- ½ cup Sprouts

- ½ cup Beetroot

- ½ cup Purple cabbage

- 4 large Collard leaves

<u>Directions</u>:

1. Get a pan and add two cups of cold water. Add the cup of quinoa and allow it to boil. When it boils, reduce the heat and let it simmer until the water is completely evaporated. Prepare the collard leaves, wash them and spread them out like a typical warp.

2. Then spread the hummus over each leaf. Cut and lay out the avocado on each leaf, from bottom to top. Spread the quinoa and each leaf. Fill the remaining ingredients.

3. Fold the leaves from bottom to top and roll in other to form regular wraps. This process will result in four wraps. So, enjoy and refrigerate the rest.

Nutrition: 119 calories 25g protein 15g fiber

Pine Nut and Garlic Sauce

Preparation & Cooking Time: 30 minutes

Servings: 2

Ingredients:

- 2 bunch Fresh basils
- 2 bunch Fresh cilantro
- 2 cups Olive oil
- 6 cloves Fresh garlic
- 1 cup Grated soybean/rice cheese parmesan style
- 2 cups Pine nuts
- Fresh pepper

Directions:

Get clean water and wash cilantro and basil. Put them in a food processor, along with the nuts. Chop for a few seconds. Finally, toss the rest ingredients in and blast until it transforms into a thick, creamy paste.

Nutrition: 151 calories 12g fiber 30g protein

Turmeric Curry and Roasted Cauliflower

Preparation & Cooking Time: 45 minutes

Servings: 4

Ingredients:

For the curry

- 1 tsp Turmeric powder
- 1 ½ cup Water
- 1 tsp Himalayan salt

- ½ tsp Garam masala

- ½ tsp Chili powder

- 2 cups Red onions

- 2 cups Cauliflowers (floret)

- ½ tsp Salt

- ½ cup Roma tomatoes

- 1 Bell pepper/capsicum

- 1 tbsp Coriander

- 2 cups Coconut milk (unsweetened

- 2 tbsp Coconut oil

- 3 cloves Garlic

- 1 tsp Ginger powder

- 1cm Turmeric (fresh)

For Masala

- 6 Cloves

- 1 tbsp Cumin seeds

- 1 ½ tbsp Coriander seeds

- 1 ¼ inch Cinnamon stick

- ½ cup Raw cashew

- Pinch Cardamom powder

Directions:

1. First of all, preheat the oven to 200°C. Get a large mixing bowl and add the powdered turmeric, coconut oil, a pinch of salt and the cauliflower.

2. Use your hands and mix them together properly. Now, get a baking tray lined with baking powder and pour the mix into it. Put it in the oven for twenty to thirty minutes.

3. Mind you, do not let the cauliflower burn. While the cauliflower is cooking in the oven, we shift our attention to the Masala. To make the Masala, blend all the masala ingredients in a food processor and make sure it is completely smooth.

4. Next, get a large pan and heat the coconut oil over a gentle heat. Add garlic, ginger, and onions and cook gently between two to three minutes. Next, add bell pepper/capsicum and tomatoes.

5. Cook until tomatoes begin to fall apart. Now add the masala mix and stir for two to three minutes. Keep stirring to avoid it from sticking or getting burnt. Once its thoroughly mixed, add chili pepper, turmeric, and coconut milk, as well as, water (as much as you desire).

6. Reduce the heat down to simmer and allow it to cook for five minutes. Season to taste. When cauliflower is done, take it away from the oven and add to the pan. Mix it thoroughly. Switch of the heat. When you decide to serve, stir through the cilantro/coriander. Serve! You can have it with brown rice or quinoa.

Nutrition: 251 calories 19g fiber 34g protein

Hearty Minestrone

Preparation & Cooking Time: 35 minutes

Servings: 2

Ingredients:

- 1 Basil

- ½ cup Carrot

- ½ cup Sweet potato

- ¼ Red onion

- 1 tbsp Coconut oil

- ½ cup Aubergine (eggplant)

- 1 cup Vegetable stock

- ½ cup Zucchini (courgette)

- 1 cup Tomato juice (fresh/bought)

- ½ cup Beans

- ½ cup Carrot

- Black pepper and Himalayan salt

Directions:

1. Wash and dice the onion and carrot. Cube the courgette, aubergine, and potato. Next fry the onion, carrot, courgette, aubergine, and potato in a large pot for two minutes.

2. Add the tomato juice, the stock, and beans. Bring it to a boil and reduce the heat to simmer for eight to ten minutes. Add the basil and stir. Season to taste.

Nutrition: 157 calories 36g protein 20g fiber

French Onion and Kale Soup

Preparation & Cooking Time: 30 minutes

Servings: 4

Ingredients:

- 1 tablespoon avocado oil

- 2 cups thinly sliced yellow onions (3 medium)

- 1 teaspoon unrefined whole cane sugar, such as Sucanat

- 1 cup vegetable broth

- 2 cups water

- 2 tablespoons coconut aminos

- 2 garlic cloves, crushed

- ½ teaspoon dried thyme

- ½ teaspoon sea salt

- 3 kale stalks, stemmed and cut into ribbons (about 2 cups)

Directions:

1. In a medium soup pot over medium-high heat, heat the avocado oil. Add the onions and sauté for 3 to 5 minutes, or until the onions begin to get soft.

2. Add the sugar and continue to sauté, stirring continuously, for 8 to 10 minutes, or until the onions are slightly caramelized.

3. Add the vegetable broth, water, coconut aminos, garlic, thyme, and salt. Reduce the heat to medium-low, and simmer for 5 to 7 minutes. Adjust seasonings, if necessary.

4. Add the kale and leave over the heat just long enough for the kale to wilt.

5. Remove from the heat, ladle into 2 large or 4 small bowls, and serve.

Nutrition: 183 calories 14g fiber 39.8g protein

Ginger-Maple Yam Casserole

Preparation & Cooking Time: *50 minutes*

Servings: *4*

Ingredients:

- 2 yams, peeled and cut into ½-inch chunks

- ¼ cup fresh ginger, peeled and grated

- 2 tbsp. avocado oil

- 2 tbsp. pure maple syrup

- 4 tsp. cardamom

- A pinch of sea salt

Directions:

1. Preheat the oven to 375F.

2. In a casserole dish, combine the yams, ginger, oil, maple syrup, cardamom, and salt. Mix well.

3. Cover and bake for 40 minutes.

4. Serve.

Nutrition: Calories: 144 Fat: 7g Carbohydrates: 20g Protein: 1g

Layered Cabbage Roll Casserole

Preparation & Cooking Time: 50 minutes

Servings: 4

Ingredients:

- 1 cup quinoa

- ½ red onion, finely chopped

- 4 garlic cloves, minced

- 4 white mushrooms, finely chopped

- 1 (28-ounce) can diced tomatoes, drained

- 2 cups low-sodium vegetable stock

- ¼ cup minced fresh basil

- 8 green cabbage leaves, whole

Directions:

1. Preheat the oven to 350F.

2. In a casserole dish, combine 2 tbsp. red onion, ¼ cup quinoa, 1 minced garlic clove, and 1 chopped mushroom. Add ¼ can of tomatoes, ½ cup stock, and 1 tbsp. basil. Stir to mix.

3. Top with 2 cabbage leaves. Repeat steps 2 and 3 until all of the ingredients are used up.

4. Cover and bake for 40 minutes.

5. Rest for 10 minutes and serve.

Nutrition: Calories: 261 Fat: 2g Carbohydrates: 51g Protein: 12g

Vegetarian Pie

Preparation & Cooking Time: 1 hour 40 minutes

Servings: 8

Ingredients:

Ingredients for topping:

- 5 cups of water

- 1¼ cups yellow cornmeal

For filing:

- 1 tbsp. extra-virgin olive oil

- 1 large onion, chopped

- 1 medium red bell pepper, seeded and chopped

- 2 garlic cloves, minced

- 1 tsp. dried oregano, crushed

- 2 tsp. chili powder

- 2 cups fresh tomatoes, chopped

- 2½ cups cooked pinto beans

- 2 cups boiled corn kernels

Directions:

1. Preheat the oven to 375 F. Lightly grease a shallow baking dish.

2. In a pan, add the water over medium-high heat and bring to a boil.

3. Slowly, add the cornmeal, stirring continuously.

4. Reduce the heat to low and cook covered for about 20 minutes, stirring occasionally.

5. Meanwhile, prepare the filling. In a large skillet, heat the oil over medium heat and sauté the onion and bell pepper for about 3-4 minutes.

6. Add the garlic, oregano, and spices and sauté for about 1 minute

7. Add the remaining ingredients and stir to combine.

8. Reduce the heat to low and simmer for about 10-15 minutes, stirring occasionally.

9. Remove from the heat.

10. Place half of the Cooked cornmeal into the Prepared baking dish evenly.

11. Place the filling mixture over the cornmeal evenly.

12. Place the remaining cornmeal over the filling mixture evenly.

13. Bake for 45-50 minutes or until the top becomes golden brown.

14. Remove the pie from the oven and set it aside for about 5 minutes before serving.

Nutrition: Calories: 350 Fat: 3.9g Carbohydrates: 58.2g Protein: 16.8g

Chapter 7: Dessert and Snacks

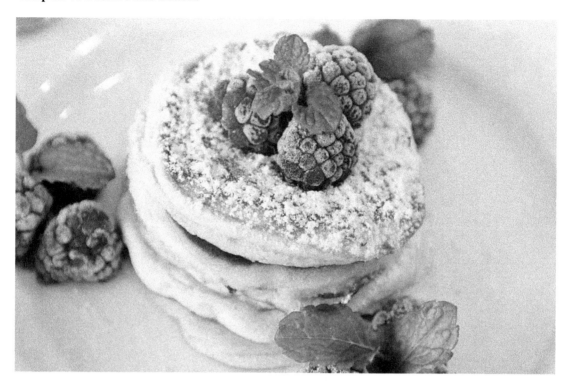

Grilled Watermelon

Preparation Cooking time: 1*4 minutes*

Servings: *4*

Ingredients

- 1 watermelon, peeled and cut into 1-inch-thick wedges

- 1 garlic clove, minced finely

- 2 tablespoons fresh key lime juice

- Pinch of cayenne powder

- Pinch of sea salt

Directions

1. Preheat the grill to high heat.

2. Grease the grill grate.

3. Place the watermelon pieces onto the grill and cook for about 2 minutes per side.

4. Meanwhile, in a bowl, mix together the remaining ingredients.

5. Drizzle the watermelon slices with garlic mixture and serve.

Nutritional Values Calories 11 Total Fat 0.1 g Total Carbs 2.7 g   Fiber 0.2 g Protein 0.2 g

Lime Sorbet

Preparation time: *10 minutes*

Servings: *4*

Ingredients

- 2 tablespoons fresh key lime zest, grated

- ½ cup agave nectar

- 2 cups spring water

- 1½ cups fresh key lime juice

Directions

1. Freeze ice cream maker tub for about 24 hours before making this sorbet.

2. In a non-stick saucepan, add all of the ingredients (except for lime juice) over medium heat and simmer for about 1 minute, stirring continuously.

3. Remove the pan of mixture from heat and stir in the lime juice.

4. Transfer this into an airtight container and refrigerate for about 2 hours.

5. Now, place the lime mixture into an ice cream maker and process it according to the manufacturer's directions.

6. Return the ice cream to the airtight container and freeze for about 2 hours.

Nutritional Values Calories 130 Total Fat 0 g Total Carbs 33.4 g Fiber 2.3 g Protein 0.1 g

Homemade Protein Bar

Preparation & Cooking Time: 15 minutes

Servings: 4

Ingredients:

- 1 cup nut butter

- 4 tablespoons coconut oil

- 2 scoops vanilla protein

- Stevia, to taste

- ½ teaspoon of sea salt

- Optional Ingredients:

- 1 teaspoon cinnamon

Directions:

1. Mix coconut oil with butter, protein, stevia, and salt in a dish.

2. Stir in cinnamon and chocolate chip.

3. Press the mixture firmly and freeze until firm.

4. Cut the crust into small bars.

5. Serve and enjoy.

Nutrition: Calories 179 Total Fat 15.7 g Saturated Fat 8 g

Total Carbs 4.8 g Sugar 3.6 g Fiber 0.8 g Sodium 43 mg Protein 5.6 g

Coconut Chip Cookies

Preparation & Cooking Time: *25 minutes*

Servings: *4*

Ingredients:

- 1 cup almond flour

- ½ cup cacao nibs

- ½ cup coconut flakes, unsweetened

- 1/3 cup erythritol

- ½ cup almond butter

- ¼ cup nut butter, melted

- ¼ cup almond milk

- Stevia, to taste

- ¼ teaspoon of sea salt

Directions:

1. Preheat your oven to 350 degrees F.

2. Layer a cookie sheet with parchment paper.

3. Add and then combine all the dry ingredients in a glass bowl.

4. Whisk in butter, almond milk, vanilla essence, stevia, and almond butter.

5. Beat well, then stir in the dry mixture. Mix well.

6. Spoon out a tablespoon of cookie dough on the cookie sheet.

7. Add more dough to make as many as 16 cookies.

8. Flatten each cookie using your fingers.

9. Bake for 25 minutes until golden brown.

10. Let them sit for 15 minutes.

11. Serve.

Nutrition: Calories 192 Total Fat 17.44 g Saturated Fat 11.5 g Cholesterol 125 mg Total Carbs 2.2 g Sugar 1.4 g Fiber 2.1 g Sodium 135 mg Protein 4.7 g

Chickpea Tofu

INGREDIENTS:

- 2 cups of spring water (or warm alkaline water)

- 1 cup of Kamut flour

- 1 teaspoon of sea salt

- 1 Parsley

STEP IN PREPARATION

STEP 1: Put all the ingredients in a saucepan and on medium-high heat. Whisk them together for 3-5 minutes till it gets a porridge-like consistency.

STEP 2: Pour this mixture into a baking dish (smoothen it with something like a spatula)

STEP 3: Allow it to cool by setting inside a refrigerator for 30 minutes until it becomes strong.

STEP 4: Bring it down and transfer onto a cutting board. Gradually slice into cubes. Serve and enjoy.

Banana Pie

INGREDIENTS:

For pie mixture, the things needed are;

- 6 bananas

- 7 Coconuts

- 1 cup of milk (walnut milk)

- 3 tablespoons of agave

- 1/8 tablespoon of sea salt

For the Crust;

- 1 ½ cup of dates

- 1 ½ cups of unsweetened coconut flakes

- ¼ cup of agave

- ¼ tablespoon of sea salt

STEPS IN PREPARATION

STEP 1: Put all the ingredients for making the crust into a blender and process for 20 minutes until it forms a ball

STEP 2: Spread out crust mixture on a parchment paper

STEP 3: place the banana sliced thinly and then store in a refrigerator

STEP 4: Add all the pie mixture ingredients to a large bowl and mix with a spoon until it is well blended, then pour pie mixture into spring form pan. Cover with foil and allow it to be set in freezer for 3 hours.

STEP 5: Remove, cool and serve.

Mango Cheese Cake

INGREDIENTS:

For the cheesecake mixture;

- 2 cups of brazil nuts

- 1 ½ cups of walnut milk

- ¼ cup of agave

- 5-6 dates

- 2 tablespoon of lime juice

- 1 tablespoon of sea moss gel

- ¼ teaspoon of sea salt

For the crust;

- 1 ½ cups of dates

- 1 ½ cups of coconut flakes

- ¼ cup of agave

- ¼ tablespoon of sea salt

STEPS IN PREPARATION

STEP 1: Assemble all the crust ingredients into a blender and process for 20 seconds. Spread the crust into a pan

STEP 2: Slice mango and place along the corners of the pan then sit in freezer

STEP 3: Add all the cheese cake mixture ingredients to blender until it is smoothened

STEP 4: Pour mixture into crust, cover with foil and allow it to set for 3-4 hours.

Avocado Gazpacho

Preparation & Cooking time: *15 minutes*

Servings: *6*

Ingredients

- 3 large avocados; peeled, pitted, and chopped

- 1/3 cup fresh cilantro leaves

- 3 cups spring water

- 2 tablespoons fresh key lime juice

- ¼ teaspoon cayenne powder

- Sea salt, as needed

Directions

1. In a high-powered blender, put all ingredients and pulse until smooth.

2. Transfer the soup into a large bowl.

3. Cover the bowl of gazpacho and refrigerate to chill for at least 2–3 hours before serving.

Nutritional Values Calories 206 Total Fat 19.6 g Total Carbs 8.8 g Fiber 6.8 g Protein 1.9 g

Chocolate Crunch Bars

Preparation & Cooking Time: 10 minutes

Servings: 4

Ingredients:

- 1 1/2 cups sugar-free chocolate chips

- 1 cup almond butter

- Stevia to taste

- 1/4 cup coconut oil

- 3 cups pecans, chopped

Directions:

1. Layer an 8-inch baking pan with parchment paper.

2. Mix chocolate chips with butter, coconut oil, and sweetener in a bowl.

3. Melt it by heating in a microwave for 2 to 3 minutes until well mixed.

4. Stir in nuts and seeds. Mix gently.

5. Pour this batter carefully into the baking pan and spread evenly.

6. Refrigerate for 2 to 3 hours.

7. Slice and serve.

Nutrition: Calories 316 Total Fat 30.9 g Total Carbs 8.3 g Sugar 1.8 g Fiber 3.8 g

Sodium 8 mg Protein 6.4 g

Shortbread Cookies

Preparation & Cooking Time: 80 minutes

Servings: 6

Ingredients:

- 2 1/2 cups almond flour

- 6 tablespoons nut butter

- 1/2 cup erythritol

- 1 teaspoon vanilla essence

Dirctions:

1. Preheat your oven to 350 degrees F.

2. Layer a cookie sheet with parchment paper.

3. Beat butter with erythritol until fluffy.

4. Stir in vanilla essence and almond flour. Mix well until becomes crumbly.

5. Spoon out a tablespoon of cookie dough onto the cookie sheet.

6. Add more dough to make as many cookies.

7. Bake for 15 minutes until brown.

8. Serve.

Nutrition: Calories 288 Total Fat 25.3 g Saturated Fat 6.7 g Cholesterol 23 mg Total Carbs 9.6 g Fiber 3.8 g Sodium 74 mg Potassium 3 mg Protein 7.6 g

Peanut Butter Bars

Preparation & *Cooking time:* 20 minutes

Servings: 6

Ingredients:

- 3/4 cup almond flour

- 2 oz. almond butter

- 1/4 cup Swerve

- 1/2 cup peanut butter

- 1/2 teaspoon vanilla

Directions:

1. Combine all the ingredients for bars.

2. Transfer this mixture to a 6-inch small pan. Press it firmly.

3. Refrigerate for 30 minutes.

4. Slice and serve.

Nutrition: Calories 214 Total Fat 19 g Saturated Fat 5.8 g Cholesterol 15 mg Total Carbs 6.5 g Sugar 1.9 g Fiber 2.1 g Sodium 123 mg Protein 6.5 g

Zucchini Bread Pancakes

Preparation & Cooking Time: 50 minutes

Servings: *3*

Ingredients:

- Grape seed oil, 1 tbsp.

- Chopped walnuts, .5 c

- Walnut milk, 2 c

- Shredded zucchini, 1 c

- Mashed burro banana, .25 c

- Date sugar, 2 tbsp.

- Kamut flour or spelt, 2 c

Directions:

1. Place the date sugar and flour into a bowl. Whisk together.

2. Add in the mashed banana and walnut milk. Stir until combined. Remember to scrape the bowl to get all the dry mixture. Add in walnuts and zucchini. Stir well until combined.

3. Place the grape seed oil onto a griddle and warm.

4. Pour .25 cup batter on the hot griddle. Leave it along until bubbles begin forming on to surface. Carefully turn over the pancake and cook another four minutes until cooked through.

5. Place the pancakes onto a serving plate and enjoy with some agave syrup.

Nutrition: Calories: 246 Carbohydrates: 49.2 g Fiber: 4.6 g Protein: 7.8 g

Chocolate Avocado Mousse

Preparation & Cooking Time: *15 minutes*

Servings: *04*

Ingredients:

- Coconut water, 2/3 cup

- Hass avocado, ½

- Raw cacao, 2 teaspoons

- Vanilla, 1 teaspoon

- Dates, three (3)

- Sea salt, one (1) teaspoon

- Dark chocolate shavings

Directions:

1. Blend all ingredients.

2. Blast until it becomes thick and smooth, as you wish.

3. Put in a fridge and allow it to get firm.

Nutrition: Calories: 181.8 Fat: 151. g Protein: 12 g

Sweet Tahini Dip with Ginger Cinnamon Fruit

Preparation & Cooking Time:15 minutes

Servings: *2*

Ingredients:

- Cinnamon, one (1) teaspoon

- Green apple, one (1)

- Pear, one (1)

- Fresh ginger, two (2) or three (3)

- Celtic sea salt, one (1) teaspoon

- Ingredients for sweet Tahini:

- Almond butter (raw), three (3) teaspoons

- Tahini (one big scoop), three (3) teaspoons

- Coconut oil, two (2) teaspoons

- Cayenne (optional), ¼ teaspoons

- Wheat-free tamari, two (2) teaspoons

- Liquid coconut nectar, one (1) teaspoon

Directions:

1. Get a clean mixing bowl.

2. Grate the ginger, add cinnamon, sea salt, and mix in the bowl.

3. Dice apple and pear into little cubes, turn into the bowl, and mix.

4. Get a mixing bowl and mix all the ingredients.

5. Then, add the sprinkle, the sweet Tahini, and dip all over the ginger cinnamon fruit.

6. Serve.

Nutrition: Calories: 109 Fat: 10.8 g Sodium: 258 mg

Alkaline Raw Pumpkin Pie

Preparation & Cooking Time: 10 minutes

Servings: 04

Ingredients:

- Ingredients for pie crust:

- Cinnamon, one (1) teaspoon

- Dates/Turkish apricots, one (1) cup

- Raw almonds, one (1) cup

- Coconut flakes (unsweetened), one (1) cup

- Ingredients for pie filling:

- Dates, six (6)

- Cinnamon, ½ teaspoon

- Nutmeg, ½ teaspoon

- Pecans (soaked overnight), one (1) cup

- Organic pumpkin Blends (12 oz.), 1 ¼ cup

- Nutmeg, ½ teaspoon

- Sea salt (Himalayan or Celtic Sea Salt), ¼ teaspoon

- Vanilla, 1 teaspoon

- Gluten-free tamari

Directions:

Directions for pie crust:

1. Get a food processor and blend all the pie crust ingredients at the same time.

2. Make sure the mixture turns oily and sticky before you stop mixing.

3. Put the mixture in a pie pan and mold against the sides and floor, to make it stick properly.

Directions for the pie filling:

1. Mix ingredients together in a blender.

2. Add the mixture to fill in the pie crust.

3. Pour some cinnamon on top.

4. Refrigerate until it's cold and then mold.

Nutrition: Calories 135 Calories from Fat 41.4. Total Fat 4.6 g Cholesterol 11.3 mg

Conclusion

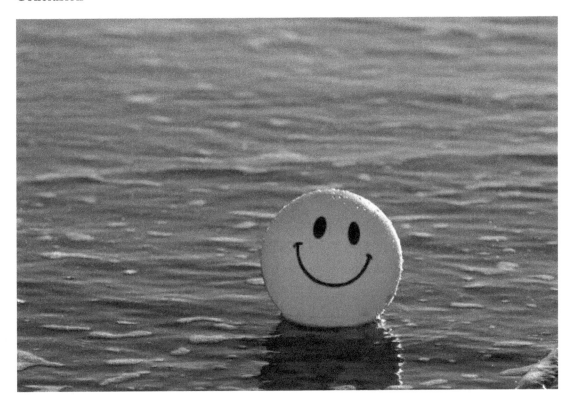

The alkaline diet is very healthy and encourages participants to eat more healthy plant foods and vegetables while restricting how you consume processed junk foods. These plants and herbs are nature's gift to man for treating several diseases and illnesses at a lesser cost than pharmaceutical drugs.

The alkaline diet is considered safe because it is all about consuming whole and unprocessed foods.

However, the healthiest diet option is one that is rich in variety. It is important to go for a diet that has a range of different grains, proteins, vitamins, vegetables, fruits, and minerals.

When you remove any single food type or group from a diet, it may make it difficult to be healthy. Although a very low protein alkaline diet can help you to lose weight, it may also increase the risk of having weak muscles and bones. Ensure to get enough protein while on the alkaline diet. Once you are sure of getting enough protein from the alkaline diet, then you can move ahead to begin this diet.

Dr. Sebi was a self-proclaimed herbalist who coined this diet. He has a questionable background and education when it comes to healing people. The diet is very restrictive and difficult to follow, even more, difficult than vegan dieting.

It can provide all the benefits that a low calorie and high fresh vegetable and fruit diet can give. The benefits are enormous, but the level of calories should wander close to the calories you burn on average, or else you will feel lethargic, and a process called cell starvation will start. However, if your main goal is to reduce weight, it can give promising results.

Trying different diets is a way to find out what type suits you. If you need fast weight loss and don't mind the restrictions, then this diet can be for you. To achieve the goals that you desire, you need to sacrifice some comforts of your life. We are used to being in bad routines because they don't require any effort. If we want to live healthily, we need to put some sort of effort and hard work into it.

The list of approved foods may not look like a lot to you, but it contains a variety of ingredients that can lead to great meals. However, if you think that you cannot handle this diet, then start the diet slowly by replacing one meal a week and then gradually improving on that.

CPSIA information can be obtained
at www.ICGtesting.com
Printed in the USA
BVHW061317220421
605633BV00007B/1479